THE
ULTIMATE
CAREGIVER
GUIDE

20 THINGS YOU MUST KNOW!

MARYANN JOHNSON, RN, MSN

Copyright © 2017 Maryann Johnson, All Rights Reserved

All rights reserved, including the rights to reproduce this book or portions thereof in any form or by any means whatsoever including electronic, mechanical, photocopying, recording, or by any information storage and retrieval system without written permission of the publisher, except for the including of brief quotations in a review.

First eBook edition September 2017

Created in the United States of America

For information about The Ultimate Caregiver Guide

Contact Author Maryann Johnson, RN, MSN

Email: Maryannj@theultimatecaregiveracademy.com

Twitter: www.twitter.com/maryannj54

Disclaimer

The purpose of this book is to encourage, educate, and entertain. Neither the author nor publisher guarantee that anyone following the techniques, suggestions, tips, ideas, or strategies will become successful. Neither author nor publisher shall have liability or responsibility to anyone with respect to loss or damage caused, or alleged to be caused, directly or indirectly, by the information contained in this book.

ISBN: 1976218349
ISBN-13:9781976218347

SYNOPSIS

With current and future trends in the healthcare field, caregivers, who are navigating complex health issues while looking after loved ones, should be educated as well. Family caregivers can face harmful impacts connected with the role, involving tiredness, loneliness and financial hardship. *The Ultimate Caregiver Guide: 20 Things You Must Know!* is an excellent resource for caregivers providing care to families, the chronically ill, and the elderly in their homes. Caregivers can help achieve families and individuals reach their optimum level of wellness and functional capability. This book will bring renewed focus, drive, assistance, relationship, and nurturing on the delivery of care.

CONTENTS

A Caregiver's Prayer	i
Introduction	1
Chapter One: What are Advance Directives?	4
Chapter Two: Types of Advance Directives	5
Chapter Three: Durable Power of Attorney for Health	6
Chapter Four: Health Care Agent	7
Chapter Five: Do Not Resuscitate Order (DNR)	9
Chapter Six: What is a Do Not Intubate (DNI) Order?	11
Chapter Seven: What is Artificial Nutrition and Hydration?	12
Chapter Eight: Skin Assessment	13
Chapter Nine: Body Mechanics	18
Chapter Ten: Gait Belt Training	22
A Nurse's Prayer	24
Chapter Eleven: Tub Bath and Showers	25
Chapter Twelve: Infection Control	29
Chapter Thirteen: Pain Management	31
Chapter Fourteen: Environment Interventions	33
Chapter Fifteen: Medical Equipment	35
Chapter Sixteen: Caregiver's Assistance	42

Chapter Seventeen: Adaptive Equipment	45
A Prayer For Caregivers	46
Chapter Eighteen: Hypertension Care	47
Chapter Nineteen: Diabetic Care	51
A Prayer for the Caregiver	59
Chapter Twenty: Alzheimer's Care	60
Resources	65
Additional Reading	66
References	67
Glossary	68
About the Author	70

A CAREGIVER'S PRAYER

Give to my heart, Lord, compassion and understanding.
Give to my hands, skills and tenderness.
Give to my ears, the ability to listen.
Give to my lips, words of comfort.
Give to me, Lord, strength for this
selfless service and enable me to
Give hope to those I am called to serve.

~Amen

INTRODUCTION

Being a caregiver is no simple assignment, nevertheless, every caregiver is the client's support system whether caring personally for a biological relative, partner, friend, neighbor, or colleague, or as a healthcare proxy or any individual supporting the elderly (aging); traumatic brain injury (TBI); physical disability (PD); human immunodeficiency virus (HIV); or acquired immune deficiency syndrome (AIDS).

Providing care also requires determining and communicating numerous goals for health care, which may include prolongment of life, alleviation of distress, or extension of time with family and friends.

> As a nurse, we have the opportunity to heal the heart, mind, soul and body of our patients, their families and ourselves. They may not remember your name but they will never forget the way you made them feel.
>
> Maya Angelou

Understanding the legal aspects of healthcare directive terminology and providing medical care independently will inform and comfort both family and caregiver as the client's condition worsens and the prognosis becomes poor. It also assists in providing appropriate clinical care at home.

Death is a natural part of life, but most of us don't feel comfortable thinking or talking about it. Taking care of a person in this situation and an individual's family means making decisions about a person's medical care when they are not able to do so. Talking with a person in this situation and their family about end-of-life medical care can help them decide what an individual wants. And when they understand a person wishes, it will be easier for them to make decisions when a person in this situation is no longer able to. It is also a good idea to put an individual's wishes in writing and make sure their family is aware of this. These actions can help a person get the kind of medical care that they want. This is especially important if their family members have different beliefs and thoughts about end-of-life care. A person in this situation has the right to accept or refuse medical care for themselves. Planning ahead and putting their wishes in writing can protect this right. Otherwise, when a person is no longer able to state what they want, their wishes might not be acted upon. Making decisions when a person is able to do so can make it easier on their family if they become very ill or injured and are not able to make decisions.

Caregivers
To the world you may be one person;
But to one person, you may be the world

~ Dr.Seuss

CHAPTER ONE

Official Preparation

What are Advance Directives?

Advance directives provide an atmosphere of respect and caring and ensure that each person's ability and right to participate in medical decision making is maximized and not compromised as a result of admission for care and treatment. They ensure that the person's wishes about his/her care, treatment and service are respected in accordance with usual and acceptable standards of practice, ethics and applicable law. The more the person, medical health personnel and community know about the purpose of advance directives and the process by which the person participates in the medical decision, the more informed and prepared everyone is. Advance directives are official legal written documents that give instructions on how a person in this situation wants to be taken care of if the individuals are too unwell to make decisions themselves. Advance directives forms are in all states and they are implemented with different types of forms and requirements.

CHAPTER TWO

Types of Advance Directives

Living Will - also called Health Care Declaration, Directive to Physicians, Health Care Directive and Medical Directive.
 These are official legal documents that point out the types of medical treatments a person in this situation should want and or doesn't want. The living will starts when a person cannot make their own decisions. A living will is a legal paper. It is a way to tell others of a person's choices for their medical care if a person cannot do so due to injury or illness. It spells out the medical care that a person in this situation wishes and does not wish to have to extend their life. For example, it may state whether or not a person wants treatment, such as breathing machines or feeding tubes. Different states have different rules about living wills and different forms to fill out. If a person in this situation should have a living will, make sure that their family and doctor know about it.

CHAPTER THREE

Durable Power of Attorney for Health Care is also referred to as Medical Power of Attorney, Power of Attorney for Health Care, Designation of Surrogate and Patient Advocate Designation.

These are official legal documents where a person should have selected an individual she trusts to make decisions about her medical care if the person are momentarily or permanently unable to communicate and make decisions for herself.

CHAPTER FOUR

Health Care Agent - also referred as the person an individual has selected as a health care representative, surrogate, health care proxy, patient advocate, and attorney-in-fact for health care.

A person in this situation should name a durable power of attorney for health care for medical decisions when an individual cannot make them yourself.

I keep my eyes always on the Lord with him at my right hand, I will not be shaken.

Psalm 16:8

CHAPTER FIVE

A **Do Not Resuscitate Order (DNR)** is a written doctor's order that prevents the medical team from starting cardiopulmonary resuscitation (CPR).

The physician is responsible for discussing DNR with the client or the client's legal representative. Appropriately signed informed consent must be obtained from the patient or legal representative. Do Not Resuscitate orders must be written and signed by the physician and remain valid as set forth in applicable local, state, and federal laws and regulations. Do Not Resuscitate orders are limited to CPR and do not include withholding of nourishment and comfort measures.

Do Not Resuscitate orders are not substitutes for advance directives. Do Not Resuscitate orders may be cancelled at any time when requested verbally or in writing by the patient or his/her legal representative. This request immediately overrides the physician's order. The medical professional staff (nurse, therapist, and social worker) contacts the physician when the client/family or legal spokespersons want to discuss Do Not Resuscitate Orders. If a decision is made by the physician to give a DNR order, the medical professional staff (nurse, therapist, or social worker) shall obtain the client's/legal spokesperson's signature on a DNR request form. The signed form is sent to the physician for signature. The order shall be effective immediately upon receipt by any hospital entity of the form signed by both the client/legal representative and physician. The original DNR order is placed in the client's medical record. The client's/legal representative's decision regarding DNR is reviewed at least every 60 days or more often if required by state, local, federal laws and regulations or by third-party payers. If the client/legal representative chooses to rescind the DNR order, the request immediately overrides the physician's order. A DNR rescind order must be obtained from the physician. The circumstances pertaining to the rescinded order are documented in the medical record.

CHAPTER SIX

What is a **Do Not Intubate (DNI)** order? A Do Not Intubate order prevents, in the event of acute or impending respiratory failure, endotracheal intubation to provide sustained assisted ventilation from being performed. Do Not Intubate, however, does not prohibit emergency management to prevent or reverse acute airway obstruction with oral, nasal or esophageal obturator airways or treatment of transient respiratory insufficiency with oxygen or a short trial of assisted ventilation with positive pressure ventilation equipment or" resuscitator" bag. DNI orders must be written and signed by the physician and remain valid as set forth in applicable local, state and federal laws and regulations. It does not substitute for advance directives, and the DNI may be rescinded at any time when requested verbally or in writing by the client or his/her legal representative. This request immediately overrides the physician's order.

CHAPTER SEVEN

What is artificial nutrition and hydration?

Artificial nutrition and hydration are treatments that allow a person to receive nutrition, meaning food, and hydration fluid when they are no longer able to take them by mouth. This treatment can be given to a person who cannot eat or drink enough to sustain life. When someone with a serious or life-limiting illness is no longer able to eat or drink, it usually means that the body is beginning to stop functioning as a result of the illness.

CHAPTER EIGHT

Skin Assessment

The development of the Braden Scale was made by Barbara Braden, PhD, RN, FAAN, and Nancy Bergstrom PhD, RN, FAAN in 1987. The Braden Scale has six categories:

1. Sensory Perception, the ability to respond meaningfully to pressure-related discomfort;
2. Moisture, the degree to which skin is exposed to moisture including incontinence (urinary or fecal), perspiration and wound drainage;
3. Activity, the degree of physical activity;
4. Mobility, the ability to change and control body position;
5. Nutrition, the usual food intake pattern; and
6. Friction/shear, which occurs when the skin moves against the support surface and is produced when adjacent surfaces slide across another.

These categories address medical situations that change tissue tolerance for pressure.

THE LAYERS OF HUMAN SKIN

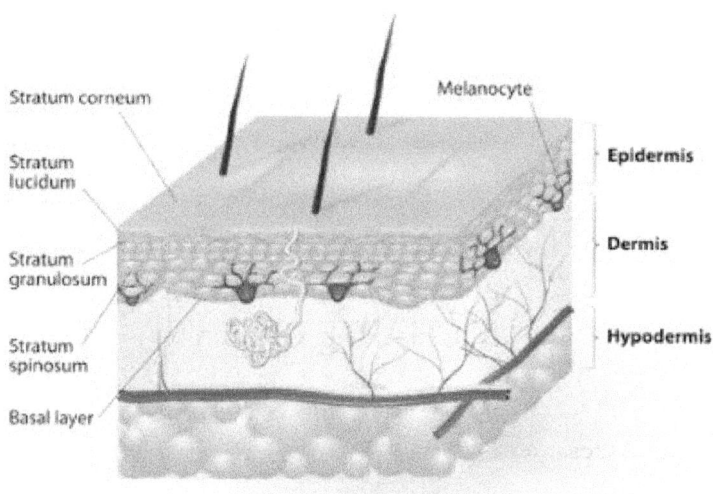

Figure 1

Skin is the largest organ in the body, an average adult has over 20 square feet of skin. Skin is the membranous barrier between an individual's outer and inner surroundings. Its three layers, the epidermis, dermis and hypodermis, protect the body against microbial and foreign substances. Careful skin assessment can be valuable in diagnosing not only skin problems, but also other systemic illness. A client's skin should be cleaned and dried after each incontinent episode using a pH balanced cleanser. Use incontinent skin barriers as needed to protect and maintain skin integrity. Select underpads, diapers, or briefs that are absorbent to wick incontinence away from the skin. Use a moisturizer on dry skin with the exception of the following areas: between the toes, groin, and under breasts. Minimize friction and shearing forces. Reposition frequently based on medical condition. Special consideration should be made for incontinence and provide interventions to minimize skin exposure. Particular attention should be paid to bony prominences and areas that remain reddened or discolored after position changes or caused by therapeutic equipment or devices.

Most pressure sores develop when you or a person you are caring for is hospitalized or confined to a chair or bed. You can take steps to prevent pressure sores. After a pressure sore has developed, you can help prevent the sore from getting worse. To prevent or help heal pressure sores:

- Minimize constant pressure, sliding across sheets or other surfaces, and slumping down in a chair or bed. You reduce the risk of pressure sores if all areas of the skin and tissue receive an adequate blood flow.
- Use pressure-relieving devices or cushions if the person you are caring for is confined to a bed or chair.
- Use a sheepskin layer or foam alternatives on chairs and beds, which reduce the incidence of new pressure sores for people older than 18 who are at risk of developing pressures sores.
- Frequently reposition the person you are caring for to help reduce the risk of developing pressure sores.
- Inspect skin daily, especially around bony areas, such as along the spine, at the lowest part of the back, around the hips, elbows and knees, and at the back of head and heels. When a pressure sore is forming, skin temperature is often warmer but can be cooler than the skin around it, and skin can feel either firmer or softer than the surrounding skin.
- Keep skin clean and free of sweat, wound drainage, urine, and feces. Use a mild cleansing soap to keep skin healthy, but be careful not to scrub the skin too hard.
- Moisturize skin with lotion, and limit exposure to dry, cold weather, because dry skin is more easily damaged.
- Do not use antiseptic solutions such as betadine or hydrogen peroxide. These can damage new and normal tissue.
- Provide good nutrition through a healthy diet with enough protein to keep skin healthy and able to heal more quickly.

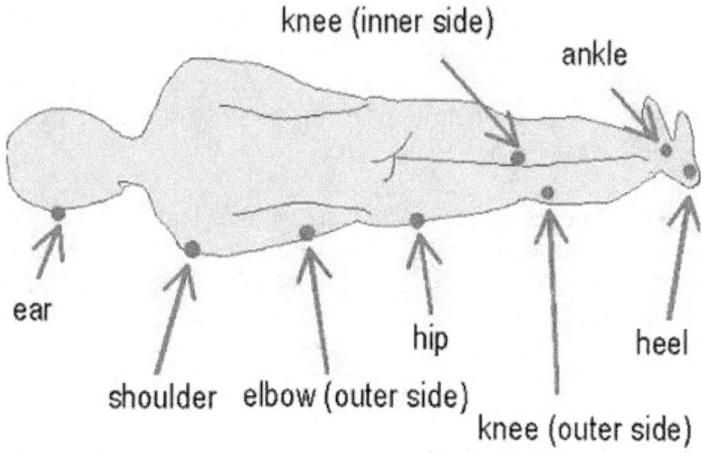

Figure 2. www.gardenrain.wordpress.com

Along with basic questions, skin history should be targeted toward the history of the present illness. The following questions assist in diagnosing skin problems:

- When exactly did it start?
- How did it start?
- How has it changed over time?
- Where else than the shown location has it spread?
- What does it feel like?
- Is there pain, itch, or any other symptoms associated with this?
- Does anything make it better or worse?
- Are there any changes in washing powder, shampoo, new pet, or personal care items?
- Are there any others in the family with same or similar symptoms?
- What medications are currently being taken or taken recently?

Here are some familiar characteristics or risk factors of skin cancer:

- Excessive sun exposure - any person who devotes substantial periods of time in the sun might develop skin cancer, mainly if the skin isn't covered. Tanning, including contact with tanning lamps and beds, increases risk.
- Fair skin - having fewer pigment cells in your skin deliver less safeguards from harmful UV radiation. If you have blond or red hair and light-colored eyes, and you freckle or sunburn effortlessly, you're much more likely to acquire skin cancer (Mayo Clinic Health letter, 2014, August. Skin Cancer, 38(8),1-3.).
- Sunny or high-altitude climates - persons who live in unclouded, hot climates are subject to additional sunlight than are individuals who reside in colder weathers. Persons living at higher altitudes, where the sunshine is greatest, are also at higher risk.

CHAPTER NINE

Body Mechanics - some client care activities require you to push, lift and carry. By using proper body mechanics, you can avoid musculoskeletal injury and fatigue and reduce the risk of injuring clients and yourself.

Proper body mechanics can be summed up in three principles:

1. Keep a low center of gravity by flexing your hips and knees instead of bending at your waist. This position distributes weight evenly between the upper and lower body and helps maintain balance.
2. Maintain a wide, stable base of support with your feet. This tactic provides lateral stability and lowers your body's center of gravity.
3. Maintain proper body alignment and keep your body's center of gravity directly over the base of support by moving your feet rather than twisting and bending at your waist.

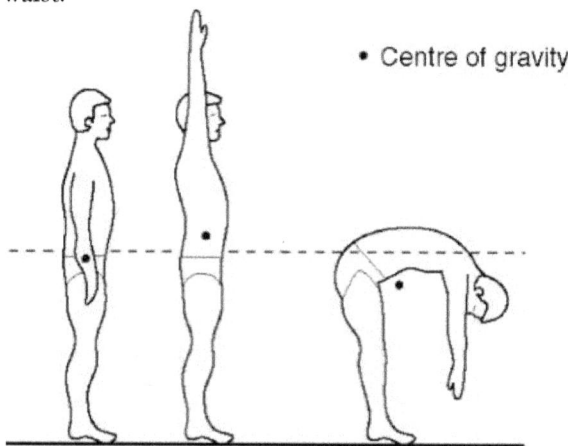

Figure 3. www.askipedia.com

Implementation of body mechanics by pushing and pulling correctly, such as:

1. Stand close to the object, with one foot slightly ahead of other, as in a walking position.
2. Tighten your leg muscles and set your pelvis by all together contracting your abdominal and gluteal muscles.
3. To push, place your hands on a stable part of the object and flex your elbows. Lean into the object by shifting weight from your back leg to your front legs and apply smooth, continuous pressure.
4. To pull, grasp the object and flex your elbows. Lean away from the object by shifting weight from your front leg to your back leg. Pull smoothly, avoiding sudden, jerky movements.
5. After you've started to move the object, keep it in motion because stopping and starting uses more energy.

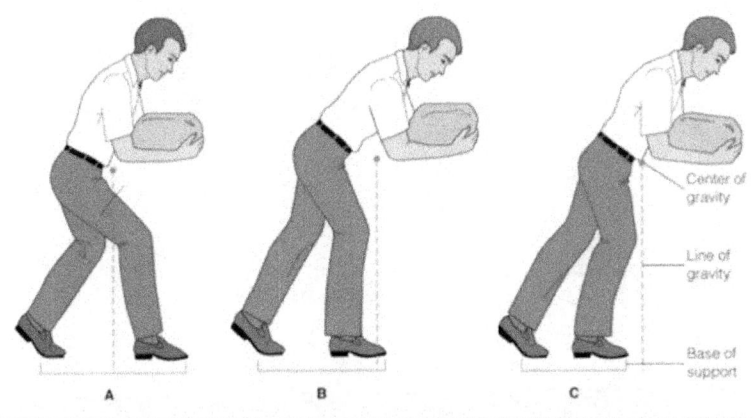

Figure 4

Implementation of body mechanics by stooping correctly:

1. Stand with your feet 10 inches to 12 inches apart and with one foot slightly ahead of the other to widen the base of support.
2. Lower yourself by flexing your knees and place more weight on your front foot than on your back foot. Keep your upper body straight by not bending at the waist.
3. To stand up again, straighten your knees and keep your back straight.

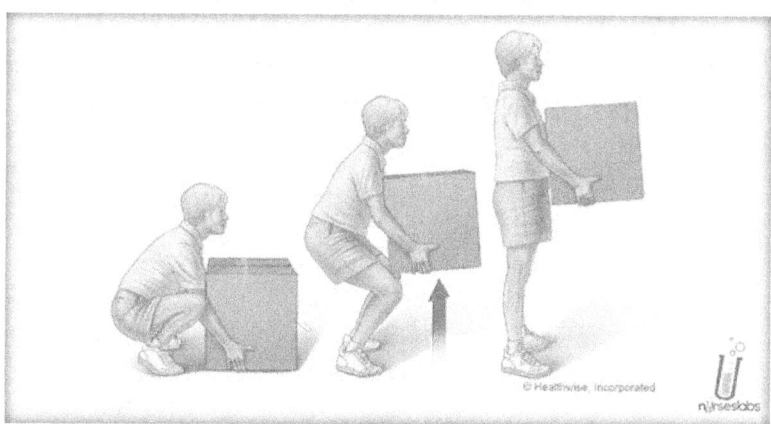

Figure 5. www.pic2fly.com

THE ULTIMATE CAREGIVER'S GUIDE: 20 THINGS YOU MUST KNOW!

<u>Implementation of body mechanics lifting and carrying correctly:</u>

1. Assume the stooping position directly in front of the object to minimize back flexion and to avoid spinal rotation when lifting.
2. Grasp the object and tighten your abdominal muscles.
3. Stand up by straightening your knees using your leg and hip muscles. Always keep your back straight to maintain a fixed center of gravity. Keep the weight of the object as close to your body as possible.
4. Carry the object close to your body at waist height near the body's center of gravity to avoid straining your back muscles.

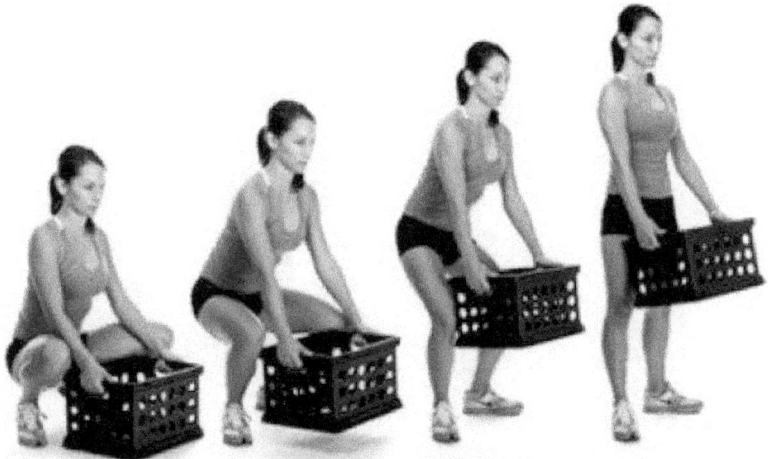

Figure 6. www.pic2fly.com

CHAPTER TEN

Gait Belt Training - before beginning ambulation, confirm that the patient does not feel light-headed. Apply a gait belt if you are unsure of the patient's stability and assist patient to a standing position. Observe his/her balance. Have the patient take a few steps while you are positioned on his/her stronger side. Grasp the walking belt in the middle of client's back.

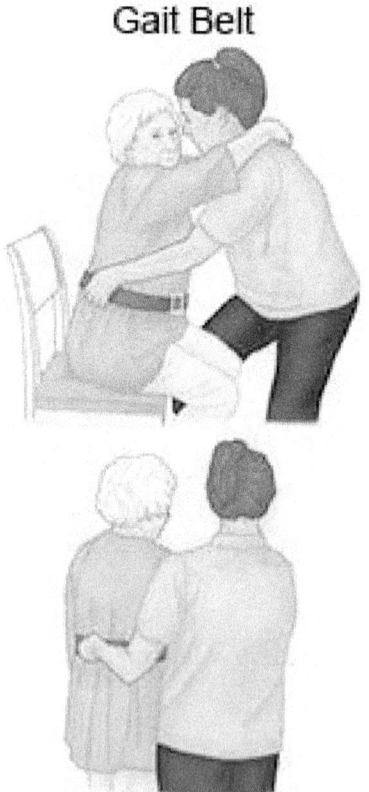

Figure 7. www.drugs.com

If the client begins to fall, gently ease him/her to the floor by holding firmly onto the gait belt, stand with feet apart to provide broad base of support, extend leg, and let client gently slide to the floor. Bend your knees to lower body as client slides to the floor.

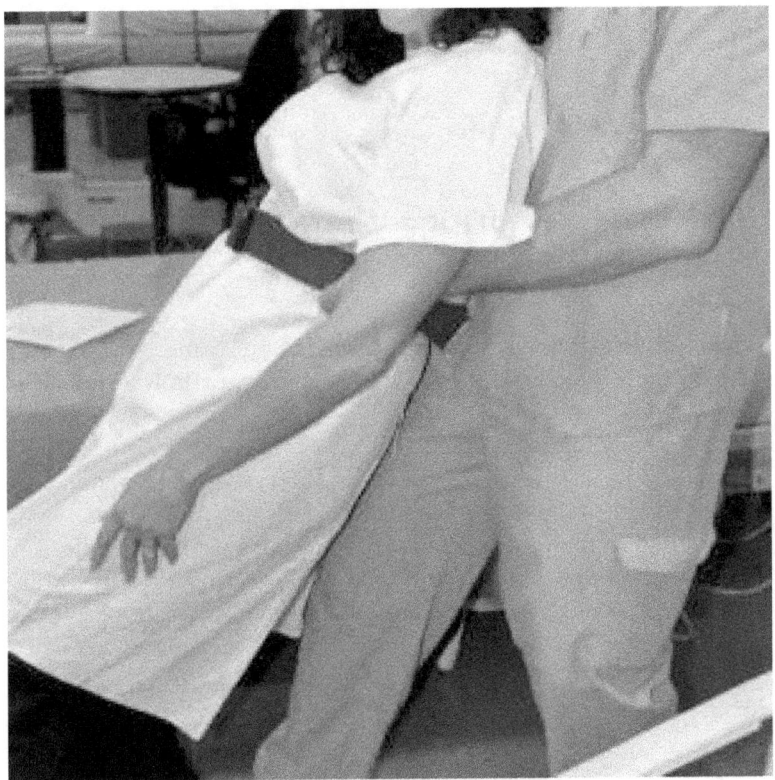

Figure 8. www.opentextbc.ca

Special considerations: Wear shoes with low heels, flexible non-slip soles, and closed backs to promote correct body alignment, smooth proper mechanics, and prevent accidents. When possible, pull, rather than push, an object because the elbow flexors are stronger than the extensors. Pulling an object also allows the use of hip and leg muscles and avoids the use of lower back muscles. When doing heavy lifting or moving, remember to use assistive or mechanical devices, if available, or obtain assistance.

A NURSE'S PRAYER
Author Unknown

O my God, teach me to receive the sick in your name.
Give to my efforts success for the glory of your holy name. It is your work!
Without you, I cannot succeed.
Grant that the sick you have placed in my care may be abundantly blessed,
and not one of them be lost because of any neglect on my part.
Help me to overcome every temporal weakness and strengthen me.
Whatever may enable me to bring joy to the lives of those I serve, give me grace, for the sake of your sick ones and those lives that will be influenced by them.
Amen.

CHAPTER ELEVEN

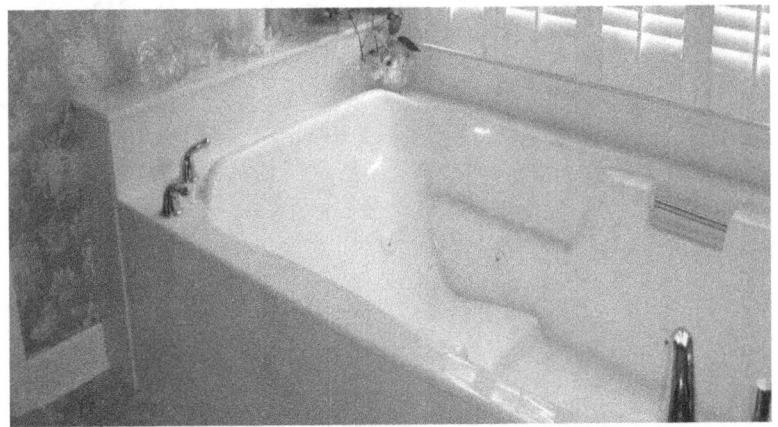

Figure 9.

Tub Bath and Showers - Tub bath and showers provide personal hygiene, stimulate circulation, and reduce tension for the patient. They also allow you to observe skin conditions and assess joint mobility and muscle strength.

1. Preparation of equipment: one or two washcloths, bath towels, skin cleanser, non skid bath mat if the tub lacks nonskid strips, non skid shower chair for shower. Prepare the bathing area before the patient arrives. Close any door

or windows and adjust the room temperature to avoid chilling the patient.

2. For a bath: Position a chair next to the tub to help the patient get in and out and to provide a seat if he or she becomes weak. Place a bath towel over the chair to cover the client if he or she becomes chilled. Place a rubber mat in the tub and fill the tub halfway with warm water and test the temperature; it should feel comfortable to the touch. Adjust water flow and temperature just before the patient gets into the tub. Place a towel mat on the floor in front of the tub to prevent slipping.

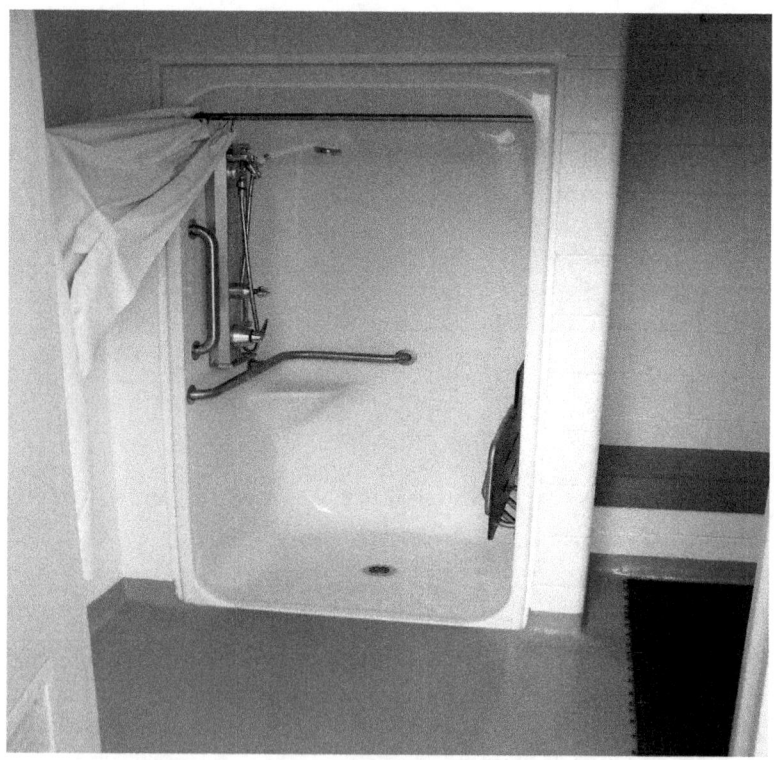

Figure 10.

3. For a shower: Place a non skid chair or shower chair in a locked position in the shower to provide support. The chair also enables the patient to sit down while washing his

or her legs and feet to reduce the risk of falling. Cover the floor of the shower with a nonskid mat unless it already has nonskid strips. Place a towel mat next to the bathing area. Adjust water flow and temperature just before the patient gets into shower. Place a rubber mat in the tub and place a towel mat on the floor in front of the shower to prevent slipping.

4. Implementation of the bath and shower: perform hand hygiene, explain the procedure to the patient, escort the patient to the bathing area, and help him or her undress, as necessary. Offer a shower cap if the patient wants to keep their hair dry, otherwise, provide shampoo. Place all items for the patient's convenience to prevent reaching and maintain his/her safety. Help the patient into the tub or shower. Encourage him or her to use handrails to prevent falling. Provide washcloths and skin cleanser, if the client has dry skin, add bath oil to water. But wait until after he gets into the tub before adding bath oil because oil makes the tub slick and increases the risk of falling. Taking care to respect the patient's privacy, help the patient bathe, as needed; cover the patient with a towel and wash beneath it to alleviate the distress of embarrassment. Be aware of signs of discomfort with bathing. If the patient is confused, don't leave him/her alone. Tell the patient to leave the door unlocked for their own safety. Stay nearby in case of an emergency and check on clients every 5 to 10 minutes.

5. Special considerations:

    a. Separate hair washing from body washing if either is distressing or overwhelming to the patient.
    b. Encourage the patient to use safety devices, bars and rails when bathing.
    c. Because bathing in warm water cause vasodilation, the client may feel faint. If so, open the tub drain or turn off the shower. Cover the patient's back with a bath towel. If the client was taking a shower, assist him/her to a chair to prevent injury

from falling.
d. If the client is able, have him/her cross their legs and tighten their thigh, abdominal, and buttock muscles, this will slow down the heart rate by doing vagal maneuver by stimulating the vagus nerve.

CHAPTER TWELVE

Infection Control - Proper removal of waste in the home provides safety and infection control for your patient, you, as well as your family.

These are steps you can follow:

1. At all times, wear disposable gloves while handling blood, other body fluids or body wastes.
2. Wash hands before and after each individual contact.
3. Wash dirty dishes in detergent and hot water right away.
4. Avoid contact with anyone who has a cold or infectious disease. Wear a mask if you have a cold or flu symptoms.
5. Keep soiled sheets, towels and clothing in a container lined with a plastic bag until laundered. Laundry should be done in hot water.
6. Wash any surfaces or equipment that have been contaminated with blood, other body fluids or body waste with soap and water, then clean with diluted household bleach using 10 parts water to 1 part bleach. Use paper towels, not reusable sponges. Again, wear disposable gloves. Put disposable items into a plastic-lined bag, then into another garbage bag. Remove gloves, making sure you do not touch the outside of the gloves with your bare hands and throw away into the second trash bag. Be certain all bags are sealed securely and dispose of them into a trash can with a close-fitting top.

7. Place all needles, syringes and connected equipment into a puncture-resistant safety sharp container or container. Needles should not be recapped, bent, removed from syringes or otherwise handled. Place the safety/sharps container in a garbage bag and then into a trash can with a tight-fitting lid.

CHAPTER THIRTEEN

Pain Management - Pain is a subjective occurrence making it challenging to describe and evaluate.

Pain is all that the suffering individual verbalizes, especially when a client self-reports pain. By medical standards, pain is classified as existence acute or chronic, being contingent on the length of symptoms.

According to Dr. J. Marsh (2013), acute pain is a result of tissue injury and resolves when the injury heals, usually in less than three months. Chronic pain is measured when it lasts more than several months beyond the expected healing time, usually more than six months. The assessment and measurement of pain strength and quality, pain character, frequency, and location duration should be suitable to the person's age. Pharmacological management of pain, including appropriate use and common side effects of drugs, is one main reason for constipation.

There are three types of primary constipation including functional constipation, slow-transit constipation, and pelvic floor dysfunction (McCance & Huether, 2014). Low-residue diet and low fluid intake are associated with functional constipation, which involves the normal rate of stool passage but difficulty with evacuation (McCance & Huether, 2014).

Women and older adults are at higher risk for constipation (WebMD, 2015). It can be caused by many different things including inadequate water and fiber intake and overuse of laxatives (WebMD, 2015).

Slow-transit constipation, involves impaired colonic motor activity with infrequent bowel movements, straining, abdominal distension, and palpable stool in the sigmoid colon (McCance & Huether, 2014). Pelvic floor dysfunction causes difficulty in expelling stool because of the inability for the muscles and anal sphincter to relax with defecation (McCance & Huether, 2014). Decreased sphincter pressure can also cause a deficit in the rectal wall elasticity, leading to constipation (Mayo Clinic, 2015).

Secondary constipation can have many origins. Some causes in older adults often come from the use of certain medications that have an impact on nerve conduction and smooth muscle functions. These medications include NSAIDs, opioids, calcium supplements and calcium antagonists (Mayo Clinic, 2015). Neurogenic disorders such as Parkinson's disease and multiple sclerosis could also be a cause, as well as certain endocrine and metabolic disorders (McCance & Huether, 2014). Constipation has the potential to cause considerable morbidity among individuals, and it can have a profound impact on personal wellbeing and quality of life (Mitchell, 2014).

Constipation is a common disorder in the elderly population. Constipation may be caused by multiple reasons. Decreased motility related to the degeneration of neurons in the mesenteric plexus, decreased neurotransmitter function, use of medications, and comorbid conditions are all possibilities for the elderly as causes of constipation (McCance & Huether, 2014).

Depression is also prevalent in the population and depressed individuals are likely to lack the motivation to eat a healthy diet and exercise (McCance & Huether, 2014). Making some lifestyle changes can often treat constipation. In that case, a diet high in fiber, plenty of water and trying to get some exercise will help relieve constipation.

In aging individuals, the advantage and disadvantage of the treatment should be measured and adjusted cautiously. Nonpharmacological pain management and consistent physical activity can reduce pain counts, increase mood, and improve functional status. Passive range of motion exercises and massage are helpful. Aging adults are less likely to state pain due to a confounded view that pain is a usual part of the advanced aging process, not wanting to inconvenience their caregivers, reasoning impairment and inadequate health knowledge.

CHAPTER FOURTEEN

Environmental interventions - Safety accidents are a major cause of injury and death, especially for people over 60. After surgery or during illness, you may be weak and less agile. A simple fall can result in a disabling injury. All clients need to take special precautions to ensure a safe living environment. Most accidents in the home can be prevented by elimination hazards.

Safety in the home suggestions:

- Emergency phone numbers are posted by each telephone.
- Lighting throughout the house is adequate.
- Electrical appliance cords are clean and in good condition. Keep the appliances away from water sources.
- An adequate number of outlets are located in each room. There are no "octopus" outlets with several plugs being used.
- Electrical outlets are grounded.
- Throw rugs have a nonskid backing and are not placed in high-traffic areas.
- Smoke detectors are in place. Batteries are checked and replaced regularly.
- Always be prepared for a sudden emergency. Be sure to have enough necessities on hand and ask family and/or friends for any help.

- Select an emergency contact to provide transportation if you need skilled medical care. Call 911 if you need emergency medical care.

Assemble a survival kit:

- Have cash (including coins) on hand to help you through the emergency period. The ATM machines and banks will not be in operation without electricity and stores will not be able to accept credit cards.
- First aid kit.
- Three days' worth of medication, including a list of the medication you take regularly and their dosages, the name of the physician prescribing it and a list of any allergies.
- List of physicians and relatives/friends who should be notified should you be injured.

CHAPTER FIFTEEN

Medical Equipment – helps provide client care and service and promotes positive client outcomes. The medical equipment company, as well as agency personnel (skilled nurse and therapist), are responsible for instructing the client/family/caregiver in the safe and effective use of medical equipment and supplies. Basic instructions should include the following, as appropriate: basic purpose, description and operating instructions, troubleshooting procedures, correct use of equipment, supplies and accessories, safety precautions and warning associated with the home use of the equipment, any necessary cleansing or disinfecting procedures of the equipment or accessories and infection control precautions, any maintenance to be performed by the patient/family caregiver, backup equipment, accessories and emergency plans, appropriate storage and transport of equipment and demonstration of the use of the equipment and return demonstration by the caregiver. The caregiver should be provided with a written checklist of equipment information and safety checks including any manufacturer's instruction for equipment with known significant safety hazards in a language and format that is reasonably understood.

Here are some practical tips on the use of an oxygen concentrator. Room air is drawn in through the felt air inlet filter on the cabinet. The air passes through dust filters, then through a special bacterial filter that traps any impurities in the air. This clean oxygen is then filtered through a special material called a "molecular sieve," which traps other gases such as nitrogen and carbon dioxide, but permits oxygen to pass through. The resulting high concentration oxygen is stored in a storage tank, which is then delivered through an adjustable flowmeter.

Front panel controls and indicators:

- Main power switch: press switch to turn unit on or off.
- Flowmeter regulates oxygen enriched air flow in liter per minute.
- Audible alarm will alarm under the following conditions: power failure, low, high cabinet temperature or air inlet filters become excessively dirty.
- Visual alarm indicators. Your unit may have individual visual alarms for any of the following conditions: power failure, dirty filters, high temperature, low battery or low system pressure. Some units have only one visual alarm called a service alarm which may light if any of the above-mentioned conditions exist.
- Hour indicator monitors total hours of usage.

Operating instructions:

- Press the main power switch to on.
- While viewing the center of the flowmeter ball, adjust the flowmeter to the flow rate prescribed by the doctor. Only use the flow setting ordered by the doctor.
- To turn your unit off, set the main power switch to the off position.
- A continuous, battery powered, audible alarm sounds if the power switch is on and an electrical power failure occurs. To shut the alarm off during power outages, press the main power switch to off.

Safety Precautions:

- No smoking.
- Do not use within six feet of a flame, glowing or burning materials.
- Do not kink or bend oxygen tubing. Do not set anything on the tubing, doing so may obstruct oxygen flow.
- Keep the unit at least six inches away from walls and

curtains. Keep the unit free from obstacles.

Cleansing and Maintenance:

- Clean the cabinet by wiping only with a damp cloth. Do not use cleaners or disinfectants that may damage the exterior surface or part.
- If you have a humidifier bottle, it should be cleaned daily as follows: wash the humidifier bottle and lid in a vinegar solution of two parts for 20 minutes. This serves as an antibacterial agent. Rinse thoroughly with fresh water and allow to air dry on its side.
- The foam air inlet filter should be cleansed by washing with soap and water and rinsing thoroughly with water. Squeeze excess water from the filter and allow to completely dry before replacing on the concentrator.

Troubleshooting:

Problem: no oxygen flow to patient, possible causes.
- Kinked or obstructed tubing.
- Leak at a connection.
- Humidifier bottle not screwed together properly after refilling, allowing oxygen to leak where it screws together. To verify flow to patient, place nosepiece in glass of water and compare bubbling to that of bubbling in humidifier bottle. They should be relatively the same. If not, recheck for loose connections.
- Check for defective nasal cannula.

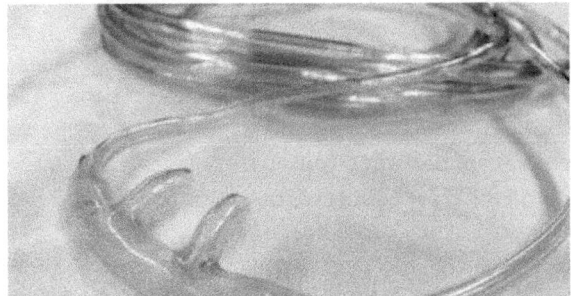

Figure 11. www.respiratory.healthcaresupply.pros.com

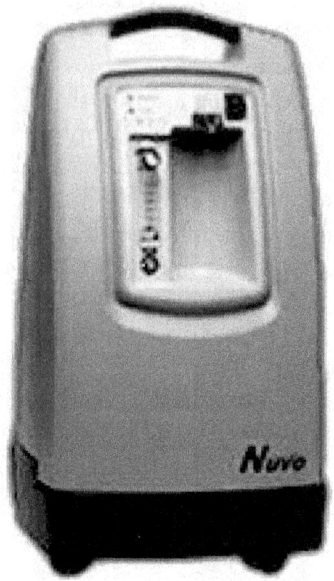

Figure 12.

Problem: Concentrator will not run. Possible causes: power failure, power cord not connected, circuit breaker activated, check all electrical connections and circuit breaker

Oxygen Safety rules: Oxygen does not explode. Oxygen does not burn by itself, but it is one of the three ingredients necessary for a fire to occur. The other two ingredients are a combustible or flammable material and a source of ignition. Prevent the chance of fire, follow these rules:

DO NOT:
- Transport oxygen in an enclosed area or the trunk of your car.
- Open cylinder valves quickly.
- Use a heavy coating of oily lotions, face creams or hair dressings while receiving oxygen.
- Use aerosol sprays in the vicinity of oxygen equipment.
- Oil or grease oxygen equipment.
- Allow oxygen tubing to be covered by any objects.

- Have oxygen on when equipment is not in use.
- Use any household electrical equipment in an oxygen-enriched atmosphere (electric razors, heaters and blankets). Keep these types of items at least five feet from your oxygen.
- Permit the use of open flames or burning tobacco in the room where oxygen is being used or stored.
- Use or handle oxygen containers roughly
- Store oxygen in a confined area
- Allow untrained persons to use or adjust any oxygen equipment.
- Attempt to fix or repair oxygen equipment.
- Store oxygen container near radiators, heat ducts, steam pipes or other sources of heat.
- Remove oxygen tanks from stand.

DO:
- Have NO SMOKING sign visible throughout the home.
- Consider having fire extinguishers available.
- Transport portable oxygen tanks in the back seat of your care and secure it properly.
- Open your window approximately one inch when transporting any oxygen equipment.

Oxygen Safeguards:
- Oxygen is a drug. The liter flow should be only that prescribed by your physician.
- Oxygen supports combustion. There should be NO SMOKING in the room when oxygen is in use.

Equipment:
- Large tank that contains 2500-2700 PSI when full.
- PSI gauge.
- Extension tubing.
- Cannula.
- Mask.

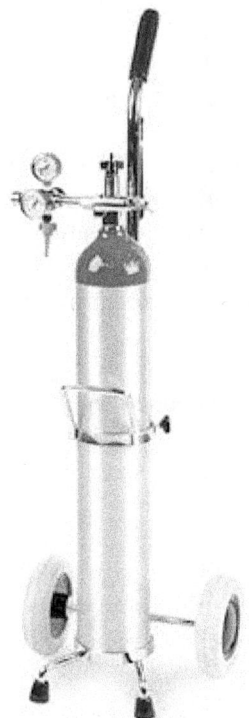

Figure 13.

Use of Oxygen:
- Open main valve on top of tank all the way and leave on at all times.
- Turn liter flow to flow rate prescribed by your physician.
- Insert prongs of cannula in the patient's nostrils. Then slide your hands along tubing lifting it up and wrapping it around the patient's ears. To finish the fit, slide adjustor up to a comfortable position under chin.

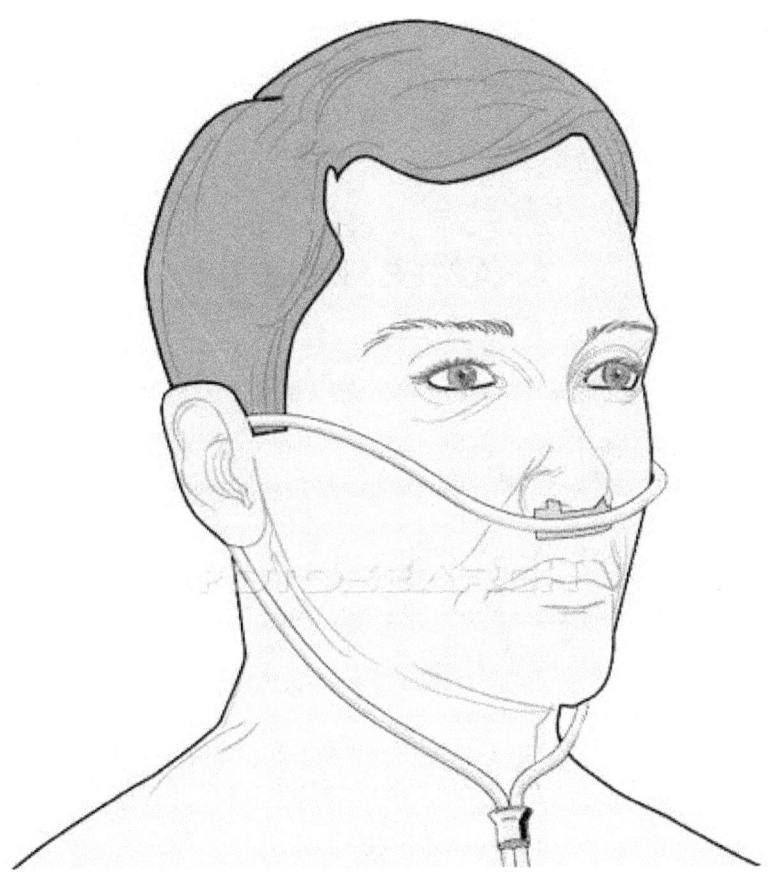

Figure 14.

CHAPTER SIXTEEN

Caregivers asking for help when caring for loved ones.

Asking for help is vital: don't attempt to do it all yourself. This can make you too worried, and you won't be capable of providing decent care. These are some helpful tips. Begin by creating a list of activities where you can use help.

1. Personal care/Activity of daily living (ADLs):
    a. Eating refers only to the act of eating itself (cutting, ability to self-feed, chewing and swallowing.
    b. Bathing includes personal hygiene tasks in the form of bathing, showering or bed baths. Can the patient manipulate faucets, regulate water temp and recognize need to bathe?
    c. Grooming —brushing of teeth and hair, application of deodorant, shaving, oral mouth care and nail care.
    d. Dressing includes the ability to choose weather-appropriate clothing and to physically put them on. Manipulate clothing fasteners and physically put on their clothes.
    e. Transferring the ability to get in/out of their place of sleep (bed, recliner and wheelchair) and self-position.

      f. Incontinence-control of bowel/bladder functions, hygiene needs, ability to use/change diaper/pads, ability to manage menstruation, ability to empty urine from a catheter bag or bedpan, colostomy/ostomy care needs.
      g. Transferring ability to get in/out of their place of sleep (bed, recliner) as well as self-positioning in bed.
2. Light housework.
3. Meals preparation.
4. Medicines (filling prescription, setting up pill box).
5. Getting supplies (clothing, toiletries, cleaning supplies, medical equipment).
6. Emotional support from family members, friends, and church members. Think of how they can help; give them a call.
7. Transportation to doctors' appointments.
8. Household maintenance (making repairs to the house, apartment, taking care of the yard).

How a Caregiver can benefit from a primary care doctor visit.

1. Write down any concerns, questions or educational needs that the client wants to ask the physician.
2. Mark the most important questions with a star ☐ and ask those questions first.
3. Make a list of the medicines that the client is taking including over-the-counter medication.
4. A caregiver should consider taking all of the client's medicines to the doctor at least once.
5. A caregiver should mark the medicines that need a new prescription with a star☐ .
6. A caregiver should ask questions about any new medicine or new treatment plan that the client's doctor prescribes for your clients such as:
      a. How will it help the clients ?
      b. Are there any risks or side effects I should know about on behalf of the client?
      c. What do I need to do for the client?

    d. Should this be written on my action plan?
7. A caregiver should ask the doctor to repeat anything that is not completely clear to them.
8. A caregiver should ask the doctor to speak slowly, use simpler words, or draw a picture to help you better understand.

CHAPTER SEVENTEEN

Adaptive Equipment - this is home care equipment that a person can use:

1. Three-in-One commode
2. Bathtub grab bars
3. Bath chairs
4. Bed rails
5. Braces
6. Chair lift
7. Grab bars, anchors
8. Home care beds
9. Hoyer lifts
10. Hydraulic lifts
11. Stand and assist lift
12. Over bed tables

A PRAYER FOR CAREGIVERS

Dear Lord,
    Being a caregiver is a full-time and exhausting task. Please bless every caregiver in a special way. Grant them grace, peace, comfort and your love as they provide care. Please send the right people at the right time to be a blessing to those caregivers who may need a break. Touch the heart of those caregivers who may need a break. Touch the hearts of those who want to help; lead and guide them in the ways that they can aid and assist. When those periods of loneliness and isolation come, please wrap loving arms around each and every caregiver and let them know that you are there.

~ Amen

CHAPTER EIGHTEEN

Hypertension/High Blood Pressure Care:

1. Understanding Hypertension

Blood pressure is the force of blood moving through your arteries. Arteries are the blood vessels that carry blood from your heart to the rest of your body. Blood pressure is measured with two numbers. The systolic pressure, the top number, measures the force of blood in your arteries when your heart contracts. The diastolic pressure, the bottom number, measures the force of blood in your arteries while your heart is relaxed/filling with blood between beats. A good blood pressure reading is when your numbers are lower or equal to 120/80; 120 is the systolic number and 80 is the diastolic number.

High blood pressure (hypertension) is when your blood pressure is usually higher than it should be. It is like a car tire with too much air in it. If the tire pressure is not lowered, there is a great risk of damage to the tire. Over time, if your high blood pressure is not lowered, there is a risk for damage to your eyes, brain, heart, blood vessels and kidneys.

There are several types of blood pressure: normal, prehypertension and high blood pressure. Normal is less than 120/80. A person should speak with their doctor if they have diabetes or kidney disease, even a small rise in either number increases the risk for heart disease and stroke.

Prehypertension is 120/80 - 140/90, which may lead to higher blood pressure. Talk with your doctor about steps you can take to lower blood pressure.

High blood pressure (hypertension) is 140/90 or higher and needs treatment. See your doctor if blood pressure is always high. High blood pressure has no symptoms, it is considered a silent condition. Over time, it can damage your heart and other organs. A person can be at risk for high blood pressure if they have the following:

- Older than 50 years.
- Overweight or obese.
- Smoke.
- Have diabetes.
- Have kidney disease.
- Hispanic or Latino/Latina.
- African American.
- A man who drinks more than one ounce of alcohol per day.
- A woman who drinks more than half an ounce of alcohol per day.
- A member of a family like their mother, father, or other relative who has high blood pressure.

2. Checking your blood pressure:

- It is important to test your blood pressure regularly.
- Keep a record of all your blood pressure readings.
- Electronic blood pressure machines rely on electronic sensors to detect the vibrations caused by the rush of blood through an artery. When the cuff is deflated, one style of blood pressure machine determines the initial burst of oscillations and translates the information into a systolic (top number for blood pressure) blood pressure reading. The diastolic (bottom number of blood pressure) measurement is made when oscillation are lowest, just before they stop. (Clinical Nursing Skills and Techniques)
- Make sure you are relaxed and comfortable. If you are anxious or uncomfortable, this will make your blood pressure rise temporarily.

- When you are taking your reading, keep still and silent. Moving and talking can affect your reading.
- Take two or three readings, each about two minutes apart, and then work out the average. Some people find that their first reading is much higher than the next reading. If this is true for you, keep taking a reading until they level out and stop falling, then use this as your reading.

3. Control hypertension in adults by using the following lifestyle modification:

- Reduce weight by maintaining normal body weight (BMI) body mass index 18.5-24.9 kg/m.
- Adopt DASH, which stands for " Dietary Approaches to Stop Hypertension' eating plan by consuming a diet rich in fruit, vegetables, and low-fat dairy products with a reduced content of saturated and total fat (http://www.nhlbi.nih.gov).
- Lower sodium intake by consuming no more than 2,400 mg of sodium/day. Further reduction of sodium intake to 1,500 mg/day is desirable since it is associated with even greater reduction in blood pressure. Reduce intake by at least 1,000 mg/day since that will lower blood pressure, even if the desired daily sodium intake is not achieved.
- Physical activity by engaging in regular aerobic physical activity such as brisk walking at least 30 minutes per day, most days of the week.
- Moderation of alcohol consumption by limiting consumption to no more than two drinks (24 oz. beer, 10 oz. wine or 3 oz. 80-proof whiskey) per day in most men, and to no more than one drink per day in women and lighter weight persons.

So, do not fear, for I am with you; do not be dismayed, for I am your god. I will strengthen you and help you; I will uphold you with my righteous right hand.

Isaiah 41:10

CHAPTER NINETEEN

Diabetic Care

1. Understanding Diabetes:
    a. Your body needs to have some sugar in the blood.
    b. Diabetes is an illness in which there is too much sugar or glucose in the blood.
    c. A blood test can determine when there is too much sugar in the blood. According to the American Diabetes Association (ADA), the following tests identify multiple ways to determine a diagnosis of diabetes:
        i. Elevated plasma glucose levels.
        ii. Fasting plasma glucose 126 mg/dl or greater.
        iii. Casual plasma glucose tolerance test 200 mg/dl or greater accompanied by classic diabetes symptoms of extreme thirst and the need to urinate often.
        iv. An oral glucose tolerance test with two-hours blood glucose of 200mg/dl or greater.
        v. Hemoglobin A1C of 6.5 % or greater.
    d. When sugar is in the blood, it moves to cells where it is used as energy. The body needs this power in the cells to endure. In order to get inside

the cells, your body needs insulin, which is made by beta cells in the pancreas.
   e. In diabetes, the blood sugar level is too high either because the pancreas is not making enough insulin to allow all the sugar to get into cells, or the insulin is not working correctly. Sometimes it is an arrangement of both.
   f. Type 1 diabetes occurs when insulin producing beta cells in the pancreas are destroyed by an autoimmune process and requires insulin, as little or no insulin is produced. Onset is acute and usually before 30 years of age and 5%-10% of the population is diagnosed with diabetes type 1.
   g. Type 2 diabetes shows decreased sensitivity to insulin (insulin resistance) and impaired beta cell function results in decreased insulin production. It is more common in persons over age 30 years and in the obese, 90%-95% of persons with diabetes are diagnosed as Type 2.
   h. If blood sugar is not appropriately controlled, it can produce health difficulties all through the body, involving damage to the nerves, kidneys, heart, feet, eyes and teeth.
   i. It is important to gain useful knowledge about the diabetes diagnosis and to understand what alters blood sugar levels. Critical plans and tools in managing diabetes are diabetes education, individual commitment, and suitable support from family, friends and providers. Knowledge of what to do is the first step.
2. Checking Blood Sugar
   a. It is important to check your blood sugar regularly. Your blood sugar levels, which can be checked using a blood glucose meter, will tell you if your blood sugar is in good control or not.
   b. All meters require a small sample of blood. Usually the easiest place to get a blood sample is from the side of a fingertip; however, it is also possible to use alternatives sites, such as your arm or palm.

i. Before the test, make sure the site is clean. Use soap and warm water to wash your hands; rub hands vigorously as you wash them. This will improve circulation, which makes it easier to get a drop of blood. Dry your hands completely.
ii. Some meters need to be coded/calibrated with each new supply of test strips. Follow the manufacturer's instructions to code your meter if needed.
iii. Do not share your meter with anyone else.
iv. Change the lancet in your lancet device each time you test your blood sugar. Use a new test strip for each test.
v. Record your numbers. Take your meter and log book with you each time you visit your health care primary care doctor.

Your doctor will tell you how often you should check your blood sugar. If you take insulin, you should check your blood sugar just before you take your insulin so that you can adjust your dose if needed. It is a good idea to check your blood sugar before you go to bed each night and first thing in the morning. Other times to test may include just before a meal and/or two hours after.

Checking before you drive can help ensure your blood sugar is safe, at least 100 mg/dl to operate a car. When you are sick, you may need to check more often. Another good rule of thumb is to test your blood sugar if you feel strange, as high and low blood sugar often have similar symptoms.

3. Short-term complications:
   - Hypoglycemia - episodes of lowered blood glucose levels. Any individual who uses insulin or oral antidiabetic medication may experience episodes of hypoglycemia periodically.
   - Hyperglycemia - episodes of high blood glucose levels. Most diabetics have some episodes of hyperglycemia. Detection and treatment are key to reducing the long-term complication of diabetes

(heart attack, blindness, and kidney failures).
- Diabetic Ketoacidosis (DKA) - Serious complications may occur which can lead to coma or death if not recognized or treated promptly. DKA may occur when a person does not have enough insulin in the blood to offset hyperglycemia, usually during illness or period of high stress.

4. Long Term Complication
   - Stroke
   - Heart disease
   - End-stage kidney disease
   - Foot/leg amputations
   - Retinopathies
   - Diabetic nephropathy
   - Diabetic neuropathy
   - Infections

5. High Blood sugar (Hyperglycemia):
   . Too much sugar in the blood is called high blood sugar or hyperglycemia. Your doctor will set your target ranges.
   a. If your blood sugar is higher than your target range, you may need adjustments in your medication, diet, activity level, or a combination of these factors.
   b. If you have noticed a trend of high blood sugars, you should contact your doctor.
   c. Illness and infection can also cause blood sugars to become too high. This is because the stress of illness and infection make the liver put extra sugar into your blood causing a higher reading.
   d. If you think a high blood sugar reading may be due to infection or illness, you need to contact your doctor right away.
   e. To prevent and treat high blood sugar, take your diabetes medication correctly every day. Your doctor will tell you if your diabetes medication is the kind you can adjust at home on your own.

    f. Exercising may help your blood sugar come down. Your doctor can give you more information on whether and when you should exercise to lower your blood sugar. In case of very high blood sugar, exercise may not be safe.
    g. Carbohydrates in foods will raise blood sugar, if your pre-meal blood sugar is already high, eating fewer carbohydrates than you normally eat may help lower it.
    h. If you have had repeated high blood sugars that are not coming down, you need to check urine ketone levels. This is done by dipping a strip into a urine sample and comparing the color of the strip into a urine sample and comparing the color of strip to the bottle. You can also measure ketone levels in the blood with certain meters, similar to how you check your blood sugar.

Symptoms of Hyperglycemia
- Trouble concentrating
- Lightheadedness
- Need to urinate often
- Extreme thirst
- Dry skin
- Blurry vision
- Slow healing wound
- Lethargy/feeling tired
- Headache

6. Low blood sugar (Hypoglycemia)
    . Blood sugar that is too low is not good for the body. Too little sugar in the blood is called hypoglycemia. Hypoglycemia is defined as blood sugar less than 70mg/dl.
    a. Low blood sugar is caused when there is more insulin in the blood than needed to balance out the sugar. This can be the result of too much of certain diabetes medications, not enough food (such as in skipping or delaying a meal) or greater-than-normal activity. Other issues like illness or

kidney problems may also cause low blood sugar.
b. Treatment for hypoglycemia is based on the rule of 15. This rule reminds a person with low blood sugar to eat or drink 15 grams of quick carbs and then recheck the blood sugar in 15 minutes. The steps should be repeated if the blood sugar is still less than 70mg/dl.
c. Some items that contain about 15 grams of quick carbs include ½ cup (4 ounces) of fruit juice or regular soda, 4 glucose tablets, 1 tube of glucose gel, about 5 pieces of hard candy or 10 jelly beans.
d. In extreme case of hypoglycemia, it is possible to become unconscious. In such cases, family or friends should not attempt to give you anything by mouth.
e. A better option is to use a glucagon kit. Glucagon is a hormone that is given by injection. It tells the liver to release stored glucose into the bloodstream. To get this kit, you need a prescription from your provider.
f. Instructions are shown in picture form on the inside of the kit, but it is a good idea to have your "support person" family member or friend look over the kit before an emergency arises.
g. If you do have to receive glucagon, you'll need a snack right afterward as the glucose from your liver may not last long. Also, be sure to refill your prescription for glucagon if you do use it, so that you will always have an emergency kit available.

Symptoms of Hypoglycemia

- Weakness
- Cold sweat/clammy feeling
- Shakiness
- Hunger
- Irritable
- Headache
- Fatigue
- Dizzy

- Fast heartbeat
- Anxious

7. Healthy Eating:
    - Meals should be spread throughout the day. It is important not to skip meals and not to "save" food servings for one big meal.
    a. You may also need a bedtime or midday snack, depending on what your provider advises and the medications you are taking.
    b. Develop the habit of reading food labels. When reading a label, focus on the total carbohydrate amount, not just sugar. A carb serving is any amount of food that contains 15 grams of carbs. This may differ from the serving size listed on the food package.
    c. Dietary fiber is a good thing for your blood sugar and overall health. Whole grains and vegetables contain fiber. The more, the better.
    d. Drink plenty of water. Beverages should be limited to sugar-free options. Avoid fruit juice, unless treating hypoglycemia. It is better to eat whole fruit instead.
    e. For a healthy weight, decrease fat intake and control portion sizes. Food is made up of three types of nutrients: carbohydrates, protein, and fat. Of these three, carbohydrates have the greatest impact on your blood sugar. Consequently, it is important to know which foods have carbohydrates and how to find their carbohydrate content on a food label.
    f. Foods, such as fruits, milk and sweets, have such high carbohydrate content, they should be eaten less often or avoided.
    g. Starches include things like bread, pasta, starchy vegetables like corn, potatoes, peas, some beans, cereal and grains.
    h. Your doctor or a dietitian can help determine the right amount of carbohydrate servings you should have at each meal. It is important to keep this

number consistent as your medication dosages may be based on you having a certain amount of carbohydrates.
i. There is no such thing as a diabetic diet. People with diabetes should eat a balanced diet of healthy foods from all the food groups.
j. Limit the use of alcohol; don't drink alcohol without eating food.

Education is the key to a diabetes management plan. An individual can reduce the risk of complications through recognition and management of symptoms by making lifestyle changes, healthy food choices, becoming more physically active, monitoring the need for medications, oral diabetes medications, and insulin injections or both.

The good news is an individual can have a "normal life" by managing and maintaining appropriate levels for the following items:

- Daily blood glucose (Pre-meal: 90-130)
- HbA1C (3-month average); less than 7%
- Cholesterol (LDL <100, HDL> 55 men, >65 women, Triglycerides <200)
- Blood Pressure < 130 systolic
- Weight
- Urine protein (microalbuminuria)

A PRAYER FOR THE CAREGIVER
By Bruce McIntyre

Unknown and often unnoticed, you are a hero nonetheless.
For your love, sacrificial, is God at his best.
You walk by faith in the darkness of the great unknown,
And your courage, even in weakness, gives life to your beloved.
You hold shaking hands and provide the ultimate care;
Your presence, the knowing, that you are simply there.
You RISE to face the giant of disease and despair,
It is your finest hour, though you may be unaware.
You are resilient, amazing, and beauty unexcelled,
You are the caregiver and you have done well.
Amen.

CHAPTER TWENTY

Alzheimer's Care

Definition of Dementia:

- A global reduction of intellectual and social functioning.
- Caused by structural damage to the brain, steady loss of memory, and how well a person can speak, think and carry on daily activities.
- A symptom of Alzheimer's disease is the most common form of dementia. (Stages of Dementia According to Medscape Nursing 1(2), 2001 Intermediate Stage Manifestation and Environmental Interventions).
- Manifestations - increasing forgetfulness, meals, medication, people, and self.
    - Environmental interventions - place food where individual can see and reach it, hand medications to the individual, and remove mirrors because a person with dementia may think that a mirror image is another person in the room.
- Manifestations - Untidiness, hoarding, and rummaging.
    - Environmental interventions - put things away as desired, do not expect individual to put them away. Provide a chest of drawers for hoarding or rummaging.

- Manifestations - Difficulty with basic activities of daily living.
    o Environmental interventions - Do for the individual what they cannot do, assess daily to know what the patient can and cannot do, allow the patient to do as much as possible. Provide assistive equipment such as a shower stool or elevated seat.
- Manifestations - Lack of insight into own behavior.
    o Environmental interventions - Do not argue or use logic; accept.a person capable of acting on or influencing each other.
- Manifestations -Wandering, becoming lost.
    o Environmental interventions - Close and perhaps lock doors on stairways and rooms that the individual should not access, fence the yard, place cues to help recognize rooms or objects, avoid physical and chemical restraints while providing areas for wandering and resting.

An individual with intermediate stages of dementia may be fearful and puzzled. Symptoms may begin slowly and increasingly get more pronounced. They could lose things, be non-responsive or preoccupied in conversation and have problems retrieving the appropriate words or even memorizing faces.

<u>Here are five pointers to enhance a patient's life with the first stages of dementia:</u>

1. Encourage them to talk about it. Let them recognize you can help them stay as self-sufficient for as long as feasible.
2. Assist them in understanding that, even with dementia, a significant and practical life is achievable.
3. Inspire individuals with the first stages of dementia to handle their daily life and physical condition. It is beneficial to consume nourishing food and be energetic.
4. End-of-life affairs need to be in order, with or without dementia.
5. Amusement and friendship has continuous benefits.

MARYANN JOHNSON, RN, MSN

How to approach communication with dementia.

Trouble with interaction can be disheartening for people with dementia and their families, so ponder resourceful ways to understand and bond with each other.

Here are six pointers to successful communication:

1. Give notice equally to spoken and unspoken signs.
2. Recognize that communication is achievable at all phases of dementia. What an individual with dementia voices or performs, or how they act has significance. Certainly, do not lose notice of the individual and whatever they are attempting to tell you.
3. Concentrate on the individual's capabilities and talents. If an individual has difficulty with speech, apply what you recognize about them and what you are sensing, which can assist in uncovering what they may be attempting to voice. Think of other methods of demonstration via music, art or additional hobbies to sustain and heighten communication.
4. Cheer up and be upbeat: Use recognizable articles to produce a feeling of relaxation and support. Encourage family to converse in ways that are familiar for them. Amusement and a sense of fun are helpful ways to benefit through strenuous stages.
5. Reunite with the individual wherever they are and put up with their different reality. If their view of reality seems puzzled, attempt to discover resourceful means around the condition rather than responding in a discouraging way. Sidestep disputing the individual or attempting to persuade them that what they consider is untrue or incorrect. A fiblet can help.
6. The term "geriatric fiblet" was coined at the 2000 World Alzheimer Congress "as necessary white lies to redirect loved ones or discourage them from detrimental behavior."

THE ULTIMATE CAREGIVER'S GUIDE: 20 THINGS YOU MUST KNOW!

<u>Ten things you can do while visiting loved ones with dementia</u>

1. Perform a hand massage with lotion.
2. Read a book, newspaper or listen to an audio book together.
3. Bring photo albums and go through pictures and reminisce.
4. Reminisce about previous events, remember a favorite vacation or family gathering when you were together.
5. Bring a balloon and toss back and forth, roll a ball from your lap to theirs or play catch.
6. Talk about Bible quotes.
7. Watch an old TV show, movie or favorite team sports.
8. Listen to favorite music.
9. Do nails, makeup and hair.
10. Bring a pet, if allowed, during the visit.

MARYANN JOHNSON, RN, MSN

Be Gentle with Those in Your Care

By
Brenda Race
1999

Did you ever wake up feeling confused and out of place?
It's not a feeling that is very nice.
Not knowing where you are or what day it would be.
Struggling with your thoughts... trying to see.

Try to imagine that feeling... never going away.
Trying to find your place every single day.
Trying so hard to remember why, and the only answer you get is a sigh.
Daylight is here, and it's not so bad, but then ... why oh, why you so sad?

No one around you seems to know.
They don't seem to know you have places to go.
If only you could find some face you knew
Just what would you do if this happened to you?

Step into my shoes for only a day.
Perhaps you will know why I run away.
What would you do if you could no longer tie your shoe?
And when it's time to dress, you don't know what to do.

What if you didn't know when or how to shower?
A task so great that perhaps you, too, would cower.
If I strike out and seem to be mean,
Perhaps it is over things that can't be seen.

Step into my shoes for only a day.
Maybe then you will see why I act this way.
So please remember as you care for me today,
To treat me with kindness and love in every way.

Be patient and tender as you guide me along my way.
Step into my shoes for only a day.

RESOURCES

American Diabetes Association
1701 North Beauregard Street
Alexandria, VA 22311
www.diabetes.org

Series of 7 booklets: Prevent Diabetes Problems
National Diabetes Information Clearinghouse
1 Information Way
Bethesda, MD 20892-3560
1-800-860-8747 or email: ndic@info.niddk.nih.gov
www.diabetes.niddk.nih.gov.

Alzheimer's Association: www.alz.org/index.asp

Eldercare locator - 1-800-677-1116 - www.eldercare.gov

What are Advance Directives?- Caringinfo:
http://www.caringinfo.org/i4a/pages/index

State-by-State Advance Directive Forms l Everplans:

https://www.everplans.com/articles/state-by-state-advance-directive-forms

ADDITIONAL READING

Leschied, Helen Grace, Alzheimer's Disease: *How One Woman Copes with her husband's illness,* Virtue, November 1988.

Mace, Nancy and Peter Rabins, MD, *The 36 Hour Day,* Johns Hopkins University Press, 2007.

REFERENCES

Mayo Clinic. (2015). Chronic constipation in older patients. Retrieved from: http://www.mayoclinic.org/medical-professionals/clinical-updates/digestive-diseases.

McCance, K. L., & Huether, S. E. (2014). *Pathophysiology: The biological basis for disease in adults and children* (7th ed.). Maryland Heights, MO: Mosby.

Mitchell, G. (2014). Managing constipation in primary care. *Primary Health Care, 24*(5), 18-22.

Web MD. (2014). Constipation Symptoms, Causes, and Diagnosis. Retrieved from: http://www.webmd.com/digestive-disorders/digestive-diseases-constipation.

High Blood Pressure Control. Retrieved from http://hyper.ahajournals.org.

Your Guide to lowering Blood Pressure. Retrieved from http://www.nhlbi.nih.gov.

Clinical Nursing Skills & Techniques. Retrieved from http://evolve.elsevier.com/Perry/Skills.

Braden Scale for predicting pressure ulcer risk. Retrieved from: https://en.wikipedia.org/wiki/Braden_Scale_for_Predicting_Pressure_Ulcer_Risk.

Mayo Clinic Health Letter 201408 Skin Cancer. Mayo Clinic Health Letter. (2014, August). Skin Cancer, *38*(8), 1-3.

"Vagal Maneuvers for a Fast Heart Rate". WebMD. 12 March 2014. Retrieved 2 March 2015.

Copstead, L & Banasik, J (2013). Pathophysiology. ed.5. Marsh, J.D., Pain (pp.959-973) St.Louis, Missouri:Saunders.

GLOSSARY

1. Advance directives- document defining the client's end-of-life care decisions.
2. Alzheimer's disease- presenile dementia, characterized by progressive confusion, memory failure, disorientation, restlessness, and speech disturbances. Cause is not fully understood.
3. Body mass index (BMI) - A measurement of weight in comparison to height. Used to categorize an individual's degree of adiposity.
4. Body mechanics- Coordinated efforts of the musculoskeletal nervous systems to maintain proper balance, posture, and body alignment.
5. Cardiac arrest- The cessation of circulating blood flow that eliminates oxygen transport or perfusion, usually precipitated by ventricular fibrillation or ventricular asystole.
6. Cardiopulmonary arrest-sudden cessation of respirations, pulse, and circulation.
7. Cardiopulmonary resuscitation (CPR)- Basic emergency procedure for life support, consisting of artificial respiration and manual external cardiac massage.
8. Center of gravity- midpoint or center of body weight.
9. Constipation- condition characterized by difficulty in passing stool or an infrequent passage of hard stool.
10. Diastolic pressure- the lower blood pressure measurement, which reflects the pressure consistently exerted within the arterial system during the period of ventricular relaxation.
11. Hypertension- condition characterized by an elevated blood pressure persistently exceeding 150/90mm Hg
12. Incontinence-inability to control urination or defecation.
13. Nasal cannula- a device for delivering oxygen by way of two small, short tubes that are inserted into the nares.
14. Pain- subjective, unpleasant sensation caused by noxious stimulation of sensory nerve endings.
15. Systolic Pressure- the higher blood pressure measurement; reflects pressure within the arterial system during the period of ventricular contraction (systole).

16. Valsalva maneuver- any forced expiratory effort against a closed airway, as when an individual holds the breath and tightens the muscles in a concerted, strenuous effort to move a heavy object or to change position in a bed.

ABOUT THE AUTHOR

Maryann Johnson was born in Chicago, Illinois. She is a disciplined, hardworking professional who exhibits dedication to the nursing profession and as a caregiver. Nursing has been her passion. She often takes care of older family members providing exceptional care. After high school, she joined the Army in 1980 and obtained licensure as a Licensed Practical Nurse (LPN). After completing an Associate degree in Nursing at Triton College, she built the foundation to further her education in nursing by obtaining a Bachelor's of Science in Nursing from Lewis University in Romeoville, Illinois and soon afterwards, earning a Master's Degree in Nursing from North Park University in Chicago, Illinois.

Johnson possesses a myriad of nursing experience ranging from clinical instructor to emergency room nursing. As an adjunct clinical instructor, her classes provided knowledge in both theory and practice, providing a positive experience. While practicing nursing, she completed a demanding curriculum in safe care including various life saving measures.

Johnson easily develops a positive rapport with clients, families, and members of the interdisciplinary team. Through excellent communication and organizational skills, she works with minimal supervision in a safe manner. She maintains open communication with clients, family, and staff permitting access to education and services to better manage the disease process. As a caregiver, Johnson enhances healthcare services access to a diverse client base.

Johnson's personal philosophy as a caregiver within the nursing field is one of great authenticity. As one gains more education and skills are fine-tuned, knowledge attainment is exponential. Her love and passion for the field of nursing and as a caregiver are exemplified by her vast nursing experiences. Becoming a registered nurse has been a personal triumph and reflects the caring nature she possesses for her patients.

*There are only four kinds of people in this world.
Those who have been caregivers, those who currently are caregivers,
those who will be caregivers, and those who will need caregivers.*

~ Rosalynn Carter

Family caregivers are a vital part of care for the elderly and chronically ill. Greater than half of family caregivers help out with a minimum of one activity of daily living and are progressively being tasked with handling challenging medical processes and equipment. *The Ultimate Caregiver Guide: 20 Things You Must Know!* assists with understanding:

- Activities of daily living.
- Importance of healthcare and end-of-life directives.
- Health and safety in the home.
- Communications with healthcare professionals.
- Assisting family members in caretaking.

Contact: Maryann Johnson RN, MSN

Maryannj@theultimatecaregiveracademy.com

Twitter: www.twitter.com/maryannj54

www.instagram.com/maryannjohnson54

Periscope: www.periscope.maryannjohnson54

Join The Ultimate Caregiver Community on Facebook

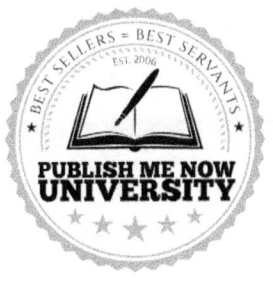

www.drfredjones.com

www.ingramcontent.com/pod-product-compliance
Lightning Source LLC
Chambersburg PA
CBHW050235230526
45470CB00005B/1968